Security for Today's Women

- ## Level of Awareness
  - ### International Travel
    - #### Parking Garages
      - Shopping Mall
        - Dorm Room
          - Socially
            - Home

*

- ## Her Daily Mindset
  - ### Her Personal Safety
    - #### Home Security
      - Self Defense
        - No Fear
          - Safe

*Written for today's women, they're smart, attractive, vibrant, career minded, multi-tasking and *distracted*?

WHY ME?

(The answers are inside)

Today's Women are always at risk on the go or at home, from the Young College Co-ed in her dorm room to the Corporate CEO in her office. Rape, Muggings and Home Invasions and murder are a growing International Problem. The nightly news used to be interesting with current world and local events, new ideas and sports. Those days are long gone. Today's news is filled with; terrorist bombs killing civilians, local shootings, drive-by shootings, home invasions, rape, drugs, sexual predators and child porn. That's just life today.

Hopefully these few pages will change your Mindset, Outlook and Life. * In some cases my grammar may suffer, correcting Your Mind-set.

DEDICATION:

This Booklet was inspired by my love for my wife. It is her desire that I offer it to you. We sincerely hope you never have cause to use this material. But, rest assured, if it is your misfortune to be attacked these responses will help you.

Your Awareness is Your Strength.

Author: Thomas Deems
Copyright©1995 – 2016 Deems

SECURITY for Today's Women

This material is graphic and written for today's women: they're smart, attractive, career minded, multi-tasking, very busy and very vulnerable to Rape, Mugging or Home invasion.

Basic self defense techniques can be applied by any Gender and at any age.
(You'll notice this booklet uses repetitive phrases and thoughts, this helps you remember it)

Your Personal Security will double or triple by increasing your awareness. Many of us are too distracted as we go about our mindless routines. We are so consumed with our cell phones, head sets, tablets, games, and sending text messages that we fail to maintain any level of "Heads-up awareness" regarding Our Own Personal Security.

This material is written in a Straight Forward, No Nonsense and often Graphic manner, because it deals with graphic events that **you and I** face every day.

Topics covered will relate to several of your daily errands including the time you spend in the security of your home or apartment.

Parents should give this booklet to their Sons and Daughters and make sure they read it, if they are leaving for school or moving away to be on their own. Rape, Robbery and Murder are in the News Daily. What if you are running 15 minutes early or 15 minutes late this morning? Could you be one of the victims in the news? Does it even matter; are you shocked to be thinking about this? Good.

You know that when we get in a rush, we forget things, we try to make-up time. We also take chances we would not normally take and that could ruin everything. For example; you parked farther away than normal so you decide to cut through the alley. Even though it's poorly lighted, wet from the rain and the trash cans are smelly, you're in a hurry, what could happen? Who are they, what do they want?

*** DATE RAPE ***

DATE RAPE:

Rape; is where the victim (Male or Female) is lured to a place under false pretense and sexually, forcibly, often brutally attacked or drugged by an individual for the purpose of their own sexual gratification. The attacker is seldom a stranger.

It does not matter if it is a friend from work, dorm occupant, or family member! Date Rape is an act of violence. If you are lucky enough to survive the attack, the first thing you must do is **Report the Attack**. The sooner the Rapist is caught the better for you and everyone else. As a witness, you are between him and prison.

Prerequisites for Rape or Date Rape;

1. You know or have seen the rapist at school, work, club, dorm or apartment.

2. They seem nice, friendly and interested in you, perhaps a little too fast?

3. Friends set you up with a date, party, dancing, day at the beach, at a bar.

4. You allow yourself to become too comfortable with someone you don't know well, it all seems so perfect, so convenient; maybe it is escalating too fast…

* The end result of Rape and Date Rape are virtually the same, most go un-reported and they are usually violent, sadistic and too often fatal.

Don't try to tell yourself that the rapist just got carried away and is sorry.

Rape is not a momentary breakdown of morals or loss of self control; it's a pre-planned act by a sick and perverse mind. Maybe you survive, will the next one?

* **Date Rape;** if you try to overlook it, saying the situation just got out of hand, you're justifying RAPE. What happens to 'your' reputation when word gets out? Is that the message you want to send?

This publication is written specifically for Women of all ages, sizes and shapes. Its intent is to make you aware of the many options you have when faced with being raped or placed in a personal attack situation. I'll also cover your options in both personal and home security. This text is expressly written to make you pay more attention to what is going on around you. Being busy is great, being too busy and oblivious to your surroundings is asking for trouble, a constant in today's world.

Congratulations on your decision to do something positive for yourself. You're reducing the chances of your being raped or attacked. Unfortunately, rape is more common today than you may realize and not just among the young. There is no age limit on rape and statistics show that a Rape of a person 10 years old and older occurs every 1.5 minutes or less, 24/7. Wisely, you have chosen to take action on your own behalf to become more aware and help inform those around you as well.

All too often people choose to look the other way, not wishing to see the unpleasant side of life, even their own. How does the thought of being the victim of rape or any other violent crime make you feel, knowing few will rush to help you? Seriously, does this make you uncomfortable, nervous or afraid? (Think about the possibility for a moment) Do you know how to re-act? Would you Re-act? You never expect to be the victim and can probably give several reasons why it couldn't happen to you. Perhaps you have already reached this conclusion. "You are just as vulnerable to being attacked as any other woman". This material will cause you to look at your lifestyle in a more realistic light. You may want to make a few simple changes to your daily routine.

As a young Marine, I learned the Marine Corps Mixed Martial Arts or the MCMMA concept. The result is a combined, condensed and more effective style, specifically tuned for "Hand to Hand combat". The Marine Corps Mixed Martial Arts (MCMMA) program also teaches a unique mind-set and it is simple, 'you are quick or you are dead'. The focus of this text is on you and your survival. These simplified techniques will teach you how to respond when being attacked, even during a rape. My "Matter of Fact" approach is simple and as lethal as you want. Hopefully, you'll learn to maintain a common sense attitude in any life threatening situation (No Panic). My concern for your safety is truly genuine. That is why in the initial portion of this book, I cover several related topics repetitiously.

This establishes the desired mindset you'll need to deal with the raw dynamics of:
1. Preventing an Attack: Constant Awareness (hint: Observe, Adapt, Overcome)
2. A Rape or Mugging: The initial Attack (Hint: Observe, Adapt, Overcome)
3. Surviving the Attack: Action & Attitude (Hint: You guessed it, OAO.)

*This next segment deals with Life Threatening Situations and should be viewed and re-viewed accordingly. My Question: How serious is your desire to live?

Those who openly prey on others are fairly obvious, usually known as bullies. You've seen them in stores, malls, shows and school; they always have the same look, the same attitudes and are usually loud with poor manners. This social group produces very few, if any rocket scientists. Now, on the other hand you have certainly noticed their counter-parts, the attractive, popular, clean-cut, very polite males or females of various ages. Now, I have described two very different types or traits within the world's population. Surely you can describe the type that is most apt to Attack you, commit a Rape, Assault & Battery, even Murder. Can you describe which type of person commits all of the above, plus home invasions? **The correct answer is NO!**

Did you know that many of those being raped know their attacker? Rape is a violent crime and not a rational act. It doesn't matter if it's a Family Member, a Friend or a Complete Stranger; it's still Rape and a criminal offense, report it! Some attackers are just thieves, it's simple they steal for a living and some are drug related. In these times of a poor economy, with high unemployment, money is scarce and some will do anything to get money, yours. Sadly, attacks should always be anticipated, even expected, anytime and anyplace. With this in mind, don't you think you should re-evaluate, even consider stepping-up your level of Awareness? Knowing Your Options, what do you think this means, how does it apply to your daily routine? You could do less walking and texting with fewer distractions, allowing you to pay attention to your surroundings.
    Increased Awareness = Decreased Danger…Less Pain…Yours!

Are You a Creature of Habit? (Below are a few hints)
* Do you usually park in the same area when you go to the; Local Food Store, Mall, Lowe's, Wal-Mart, Starbucks, Book Store, Bank, School or your apartment?
* Do you enter and exit the same way the majority of the time?
* Do you leave the check-out counter area before putting your wallet away?
* Did you look around before you left the security of the Store or Mall?

Most of us do nearly everything out of habit and it's that predictability an attacker is counting on. The elements of time, place and surprise are on the attacker's side. An attacker can select a spot and just wait; sooner or later someone will wander by. They can either take advantage of them or wait for an easier victim. (Possibly you) It could be that path through the shrubs that saves you time walking to your car. The shortcut you always take to your next class or your favorite shop, what-ever. Perhaps you make a habit of cutting down the alley between buildings when going to lunch. **WAIT! Is it isolated? So are you...Will you be found in a dumpster?**

Parking

When you enter a parking garage do you ever really notice the other cars? Are they occupied, are there people just standing around, are any of them watching you? What is the lighting like in the area you are parking? How far is it to the elevator, the door, other people or the public area? Do you see any families or sources of assistance should you need Help? If the situation strikes you as odd *Duh*, Park somewhere else. Somewhere Safer...

The Wrong way;

Alright, now you've found a good parking place. You're safely parked, you roll up the windows, gather your purse, umbrella and the two large packages you are going to return to Macy's, you open the door. As you put your foot out, you make a final check of your make-up in the rear view mirror and you need lip stick. You pause to re-apply, now it looks fine. You quickly turn to get out of the car and you are knocked unconscious. As you regain consciousness, you realize you are lying in the trunk of a car, no, wait it's your car. You're bound hand and foot with tape over your eyes and mouth. You're still groggy, but, you realize your clothes have been torn off and it feels like you've been raped. The Rapist had been quietly watching as you parked your car and gathered your large bags. Moving closer as you adjusted your make-up. He decided that you have everything he's ever wanted. You weren't paying attention and now you'll pay the ultimate price. Not paying attention will get you on TV, the evening news and a well written obituary.

The Right way;

Check the area before you get out of your *locked* car. I'm sure you've heard that before. It might pay you to pay more attention to who, what and where you are! When you get out of the car, don't hesitate. You are vulnerable when you are isolated. Move quickly to a safer, more populated area. Try to get into a habit of staying as close as possible to a busier portion of the parking garage, parking lots.

Don't stop for any reason, not to answer any questions, for example; (Got any change? What time is it? Excuse me? Use your own judgment in this area, but, don't set yourself up to be attacked). Ask yourself; am I too far from the elevator or too far from the crowd? Don't hesitate to yell for the couple ahead to "Hold the Elevator, Please". The thought of my wife waiting for a slow elevator in a dimly lit, nearly deserted parking garage drives me crazy.

Leaving the Mall or Shops

The other extreme is: Don't just walk out into the parking area with your head in your bag or anywhere else, be alert, where's your car? Care enough about your safety to at least look at the parking area, before the door shuts and possibly locks behind you. If you see the parking area is dark or deserted, Stop! Go back in and ask Mall security for an escort to your car. Many Malls provide this service, but you must ask. If you are too shy to ask or don't want to be a bother just make up a sign to wear: **Willing Victim, No questions asked, hurt me, I won't tell!**

You must pay attention to what is going on around you. We are talking about how to prevent being **Raped, Mugged or Murdered**. If you feel this subject is too serious for you, visit a Rape crisis center they'll explain the Reality. Remember, **anyplace & anytime** are where and when you have to be aware of your surroundings and be ready to react. It's time for you to wake-up and realize what is going on around you. Have you ever had the feeling you weren't alone or you're being watched, but couldn't see anybody? (Listen to your Senses) The **"Fight or Flight"** feeling is not uncommon when we find ourselves in a strange situation. The body produces an abundance of adrenalin when we're afraid or anxious. This enables us to respond with the energy needed, when attacked. (If you are trapped you'll have to Fight for your life, if you can run away do it and be quick about it.) If you think; I can't run, I'm wearing my favorite shoes…Really! Lose the shoes. These days, drug use plays a large part in the rise in thefts, attacks, including rapes. There are more and more people turning to drugs and alcohol because of the loss of their jobs, homeless due to foreclosures and the poor economy, some are thieves.

Many of those who are able to find work aren't earning enough support their lifestyle. The result is depression, more drugs and alcohol to ease the pain of reality. If people can't find a way to earn a living they soon adapt to other ways of obtaining what they want. The easy way is to steal it. The cost of drugs, crack and whatever else they can find is not that much, $5, $10, $20 per high. It's the short duration of their high and the pain of the depressed that drives them to steal.

They are not looking for a job to support their habit; they're looking for easy money, a "Target of Opportunity". The only person that can decide it won't Be your money, is you. If this line of thought makes you uneasy, then do something about it. Perhaps you should start to pay more attention to the situations you place yourself in every day. If you are in the elevator, stay near the control panel, find the alarm button. Don't hesitate for a second to hit it, even if it turns out to be a false alarm, No harm done, especially not to you. Decide now if you are willing to be a victim or are you going to maintain a higher level of Awareness. Everyone has heard the phrase, **"He who hesitates is lost".** When distracted, your head is in your bag or you're sending some useless text, you are most vulnerable.

Home Security
Another area where your attitude and aptitude are probably too relaxed is your personal security while at home. You should feel safe and secure in your home or apartment because it's your private place. Think about this, how often do you leave your doors unlocked while you go about your daily routine? How about while you were raking leaves in the backyard? If you live in an apartment, do you ever run down to the car? Maybe you go to the mailbox, the basement for your laundry or to the storage room? In any case, did you lock the door each and every time? **I know, you were only gone a minute or two. Great excuse, are you betting your life on your lame logic? Yes!**

Then there was that cute guy, who asked if the cute little kitten he was holding belonged to you…Were you Alone, Did you have any type of protection with you? Really, by protection, I meant; Pepper spray, mace, a stick, a cane, a ball point pen, nothing. If you think this is being too cautious, (again) would you bet your life on it? (If you've done these or similar things, you have been betting your life). What makes you think someone couldn't casually enter your house, walk into your bathroom and just quietly wait for you, as if there's no hurry?

Are you so sure that it couldn't happen? Does a Rapist have to brake-in or it doesn't count, are there any rules? What if they are already in your house, how would you know? **It is a Fact; most Thieves and Rapists enter through unlocked doors.**
Some of us live in secure neighborhoods behind locked gates with security guards. **But, are you really safe?** Don't be absurd. All that means is you won't be Raped by a *complete* stranger. Don't bet your life on an assumption, get-up and go lock the door and check the windows while you're at it. At least secure the window in a partially open position.

Remember, the thief or rapist is looking for an easy victim. Some will even knock on your door to see if you're home, some don't care. How good is that $2 dollar lock and what's your life worth to you? If you forget your keys all of the time, wear one on a neck chain and tuck it in your bra.

* Increasing your Awareness and developing a more positive security attitude will protect your most valuable possession, your life.

"I have nothing worth stealing"
Have you ever said that or heard others say it? Sure, we've all heard it. Here's the point I'm trying to make…Any thief will be the judge of that. If a crack head need $5; do you have anything worth $5? Here's another question; have you heard of the law of "Supply and Demand"? Did you know that as the victim you are part of the supply and demand concept? The addict's body demands a dope, the addict demands money, **as the Victim, You supply $$$ or your Life, maybe both…** Do you have anything that can be pawned for $2, 3 or $20? You bet you do! So, do you think you qualify as a potential victim? What if you don't have enough money? What if it's not money he's after, maybe he just wants you to experiment on or weird satirical sex, then what? You decide. **Remember Fight or Flight!**

Physical Size
When it comes down to it size is very important. Where would we be without it? Very few of us are built the same or have the same abilities as athletes seen on TV. So, you'll have to learn to use what you were born with and anything you can pick-up along the way. (A Stick or a Brick would be a good pick - sorry)

Most of us have heard the **"Big Bad Wolf" story.** You know, He's bigger and meaner than the pigs, therefore he wins. **Wrong Response!!** Size has very little to do with any win or lose, live or die situations. Most of us have watched in amazement as the small house cat, routes the neighbor's large dog with his tail tucked tightly between his legs. When the attacker decides the rewards aren't worth the pain and effort it will cost to achieve them, it's over. That is what you are going to convey to any would be attacker. All it takes is a tiny bit of doubt in their little mind and they'll turn tail and run. If you can cause them to think twice they'll quickly decide it's best to look somewhere else for an easier target.

Don't ever buy into any verbal abuse, it's a trick to confuse you and get you to lower your guard. When the attacker becomes convinced you won't be as easy as expected, they'll leave you alone. (This is your signal to quickly leave the area) You could be like my 105 lb mother at 70; she has the security mindset of a USMC/MMA Champion. You have the tools to cause serious pain to the largest Male or Female attacker, just using your own body parts. The mindset or attitude will be there as well, but you must work at it and you must apply yourself.

We will begin to cover the various things you can do to this creep in a few minutes. First you have to take a moment and decide if you are going to make a serious commitment to yourself. This question is very simple:
Can you find the inner strength to do *whatever it takes* to save your own life?
*You must be willing to risk it all, to save your own life.
*You must believe you can learn and practice a few simple self defense moves.
*The Truth of the matter is; if you don't think you can do it, you won't.
That's too bad, you'll lose…

Fight or Flight
You've felt this from time to time your body responds with the adrenalin needed in an emergency, I briefly spoke of this earlier. You've heard the stories of people who do amazing physical fetes. Mothers lift heavy objects off trapped loved ones in hurricanes. That's how strong the effects of adrenalin can be and you can use it to save your life.

When you are in an emergency situation use that adrenalin rush to control the situation, use its power to act. You shouldn't rush an armed attacker or try to wrestle a knife from a robber. You use your mind to think, control yourself and wait for or create your opportunity to get away. If that means you escape, do it… If it means you fight, get serious about wanting to live. Chances are your attacker won't be willing to match your courage or bet it all. Mindset; Over my dead body!

Accustomed to the nicer side of life, like family, friends, career and all of the good things? It is important that you remember there is a darker side to life and unfortunately several angry people live there. Your survival depends upon how quickly you respond or if you respond at all when confronted. If you panic, you lose control and automatically forfeit the spoils to your attacker.

To be scared and confused is a natural response. But, you must keep things in perspective, calm yourself down and think.
(If you believe you are helpless, you will be and that won't help you at all). If you freeze, you'll be beaten, raped or worse…maybe dead.

You have reached the point where I want you to think of the parts of your body, you can list as weapons. How would you best use them?

Try to name a few before leaving this page...

1.

2.

3.

4.

5.

6.

7.

8.

*Can you think of anymore?

NOTES:

Basic Self Defense Tools & Their Usage

These are the Basic Self Defense Tools & Their Usage. They are very effective, and easy to use in your defense. Your mind-set is; do I want to live or die.

Here is a list of Truly Natural Weapons which have been saving the lives of man since the beginning of time and will serve your purpose well, if you use them.

Brain   - Control Fear, Plan, Confuse them, Cause Action, Cause Pain, Escape

Fist   - Punching, Hammering

Thumbs   - Gouging, Grasping

Hands   - Gouging, Grasping, Griping, Chop, Cupped, Slap to the Ear drum

Fingers   - Gouging, Grasping, Griping, Poking

Finger Nails - Poking, Clawing and Cause pain

Elbows   - Smashing, Breaking, short inside Punch to face, temple or crotch

Knees   - Smashing, Breaking, Crushing, Attack the Groin or Face

Feet   - Kicking, Stomping, Smashing, Breaking, Pushing

Heels   - Smashing, Breaking, Think of their Throat as a target

Head   - Butting (Forward & Back), Smashing, Breaking and Escape

Teeth   - Biting, Crushing, Ripping, Holding

Any of these can be used to disable an attacker. Each of the body parts on this listed is found on each of us, from the 90 year old Grandmother, to the Martial Arts expert. Most of us rarely, if ever think of our body parts as weapons or tools for our own defense. That's if we ever think of self defense at all, until it's too late.

Your first and most important weapon is your Brain, use it to remain calm and form a plan, confuse the attacker and then when you see your chance, react. If you panic, it's simple, you lose everything. It takes serious thought to keep calm when faced with a violent situation. Make a conscious effort to look for an opportunity to escape. When you see a chance to escape use every tool or weapon you have to make it happen. Some victims are too scared to think; therefore they hesitate or don't react at all. What more could a Rapist ask for than a victim, frozen with fear and easy prey for the taking.

As distasteful as this may sound, it comes down to how strong is your desire to live? Are you one of those who believe Violence is uncivilized? If you hold that conviction too long, you'll pay the ultimate price. It never fails to amaze me, when the subject of defending yourself (against an attacker or a would-be rapist) comes up; someone is always against using violence. Don't they understand **Rape is one of the purest forms of violence?** It's as if, it is against some religious or moral code to fight for your life, using **Deadly Force** if it comes down to it. The phrases go something like this; "I don't believe in hurting anyone" or "It's too ugly to even think about taking another person's life, even to save my own". Well, Then you should think about death and being mutilated in the process. Maybe if you find the nearest Rape Clinic, volunteering will help you wake up, from your fantasy world.

Today every woman that exists is at risk. Even you, But you are not as much at risk, because you're reading this book? And taking the initiative to learn what you can do in your own defense. I'm not trying to scare you; reality should have already done that. My goal is to break through the teachings of many passive generations. Women have been raped and ravaged since the beginning of time. Why? Because society allows it, excuses range from; "Stress in the work place", or Competition is too tough, can't find work or I drank too much. The truth is more like "being one of life's marginal performers, I thought you would be an easy target". Some believe they can get drunk or high and do as they please with *their woman*, Wrong.

Note: You do know that a Rapist doesn't have to be the opposite sex, right?

For a few years I worked with Drug and Alcohol abusers in the Military. I tried to help them get sober; their families were often abused physically and mentally. I also worked with family members who were battered and abused by people who refused to acknowledge they had a problem. Many of those who were abused told me, that it was their own fault they were abused. It was often difficult to tell which were the sicker, the abused enabler or the drunken or drugged-up abuser.

A distinct sign of severe abuse is when the abused individual appears to panic, or cower when in presence of the abuser. That is the time for intervention by the authorities, a trained professional or family member. The first step is similar to the one you're taking, learning how to say "No More" and mean it. Reading this material is the first step to putting your mind on the right track to self esteem, self worth and a happier way of life, one without fear. The key is to start believing in something special, how about believing in yourself? The best thing you can do is read this book, then read it and practice some of the defensive moves with a few friends, everyone wins. You'll be surprised how many do not have your mind-set, nor do they know how to use this material. You may be saving someone else's life.

Finally, we have reached the best part: my favorite part, the laying-on of hands.

Abusing Your Attacker
From this point the material will be more graphic, because life is graphic.

You'll learn the areas of the body that you now consider to be Target Areas. It does not matter if the attacker is Male or female (OK, some parts will be different). Your objective is to survive the attack, Right? By surviving, I mean escaping by whatever means necessary.

<u>Target Areas</u>

*As you know, the following is going to get Graphic and Violent. But, if you protect yourself from being Attacked, Raped, Brutalized, even Sodomized, it's time to get Graphic. For the last time; are ready to Fight for your life? You better be!

Remember: If you don't think you Can, You Won't. But, If You Believe You Can, You Will!

Target Areas

Eyes: **Don't claw!** With a *Finger* or *Thumb*, you'll *poke* in a thrusting motion, **sharply between the eyeball and the nose.** Example: The **Thumb** on the *Right* hand will address the attackers *Left* eyeball. You are going to thrust with your *Right thumb*, so your fingers are along the attackers *Left Temple…*Look at your Right hand. Bring your thumb around to your left eye, Notice where your fingers are headed. Your reaction will thrust your thumb(s) into the eye socket(s), the eyeball will literally "POP "out, into your hand. What you do with it is up to you. I'd hold it in front of the other eye and POP it. If you decide to be a screaming, scratching and crying Victim, you'll easily be quieted by your attacker. But, if you poke your attacker's eye out, you'll quickly be turned loose. The Police will easily find the Rapist and he'll be halfway looking for them and medical attention.

Ears: Example, Take your Thumb & Fore Finger and using your finger nails, pinch your ear lobe, gently! That is called real **pain.** You're going to use that (Pure) Pain to set yourself Free. You can use your Finger & Thumb or your Teeth whichever is in the right spot at the time. **Now, when I say use them, I mean use everything, as if you are fighting for your Life, because, actually, you are.** The ear is also **easy to Remove or rip**. You *grasp* the lobe firmly with your Hand or Teeth and with a quick, upward jerk rip it off. (Upwards towards the top of the attackers head) The Ear will also sever with a strong bite. The same force as biting a carrot in half should do the trick. This applies to the nose, fingers and??

** If this subject is too extreme for your over sensitive pacifistic nature or it challenges your over developed sense of fair play, then your goodness will surely be rewarded. Maybe, just maybe you'll be found, cut open like a fish or maybe not found at all…So Wake up! You don't have time to play the helpless little girl or boy routine. You're in the real world and those who leave witnesses to Rape go to prison. So, maybe you'll find this material has the information you need to save your own life.

Nose: The Nose can be removed in the same manner as the Ear. You can do this using the *Bowling Ball Grip from behind.* Another way to stop the attack (permanently) Strike the tip of the Nose with the heel of the hand or fist, in a forceful downward motion toward the chin, then a second straight motion to push the tip of the Nose towards the eyebrows. This is a **Death Blow** if done correctly. The nose bone is first severed, then with the second movement it is driven into the Brain. (This maybe a life or Death attack and now it's strictly your decision to use it or not). You will not have a lot of time to decide what to do, But, Do Something.

Note: **The Teeth of a Human are serious weapons. You have the power to bite off anything you can get between them… Did you hear me? Anything… It's time to give it a lot of thought. So, learn this just in case, hopefully you never need it. The Nose should be considered a **Major Target.** In the event you find yourself wrestling with the attacker, just knowing you have the ability to tear or bite off the Nose or Ear. Remember, the same force used to bite a carrot in half. This will give you the edge. A Rearward head butt is also killer move as well.

Target: Adams Apple

The Adams Apple will crush easily with a forceful blow from the Fist, Edge of the Hand (a Judo Chop), Spear Thrust (Flat Hand Fingers Straight Nails lead) Kick, Elbow or Forearm. A Very Effective, Favorite is to grasp the Adams Apple with either hand, digging-in your fingers and thumb around the Adams apple, using the force you would use if you slipped on the stairs and grasped the banister so you wouldn't fall. (Power Grip) Then, **Crush it like a soda can** or ice cream cone; it has the same amount of resistance. **You should use the same amount of regard when dealing with the Attacker, as they show you, NONE!** A Forceful blow, hit, poke or chop to the Adams Apple will cause temporary paralysis to the breathing and that means, You Run Away.

Situation: **You are grabbed from behind** with your arms at your sides. Remember, don't panic, I know you'll be afraid, but, you can really cause this jerk some intense pain. Here are just a few of your options:

Thrust back with your head, target the nose. You will have to hit it the first shot, so put all you have into it. After you've broken his nose, keep it up until you are turned loose.

If you're Free, Run! If not, don't stop fighting, then fight some more!

Tip; Act as if you're going to faint. Relax and bend your knees enough to slump, make the attacker lean forward over you. Then, when you feel his head is centered above your head, spring upward as hard as you can (Imagine being at the bottom of the pool, deep end, no air, now, push hard for the surface). This should catch him off guard and do the trick, breaking his nose. (**If you're free, run for help**)

Starting your Harley, You've seen the old movies where the guy jumps on the kick starter of the old Harley. Well that same motion can set you free from this hold. You Raise Your Strongest foot as high as you can and drive your heel into the arch (Top) of their foot. As fast, hard and often as necessary to get free of the grip. The bones of the foot are not designed to take pressure from this angle, they will break. Do not feel sorry for this jerk, if you hurt him or her, so what; **you're free, and alive.**

Mind-Set Check: **Maybe the plan is to kill you after He, She or They are done raping and torturing you. So, why would you place any limits on how fiercely you respond? They're playing for keeps and you'd better be!**

Another response to being held from behind, your arms are held at your sides. (Practice these moves with a friend, gently). This must be done in a full force fluid or non-stop Motion. Shift your hips to either side; how you're being held will dictate which side is easier. At the same time, make a tight fist, your arm must remain straight; (stiff) imagine a Hammer swinging from your elbow to your knuckles. As you visualize pounding wildly on your desk, that part of your fist will smash into the crotch of the attacker. Here's the entire move: Shift your hips to either side, your fist is aligned with the attacker's crotch. Make your hammer fist and swing your arm with ALL, of your might. If you can't swing your arms, reach back and grab a handful of the attacker's crotch. Don't, in any way be gentle; this is your door to Freedom, Jerk it fast and hard. Escape, run out of the house clothes or not, you're alive, run!

Note: The nerve under your nose is extremely sensitive and you should practice attacking it. Show or teach your friends how they could use it to stop an attack or protect themselves from being bullied by anyone.

Head Butt: If you're face to face and your head is aligned with his, what are you going to do? You're going to deliver the hardest Head Butt you can. ***The head butt starts as you launch up forcefully, from your heels to the top of your head, striking their face with your hairline.*** (or where it used to be, oh sorry). Some of you think that the head butt will hurt you, not as much as it will hurt the attacker. Try these examples as I describe them; with your fingernail, press the sharp edge to the following points on your face, be serious, but try not to scar yourself.

A strong Head Butt will cut or split the skin where it covers the bones of the face:

1. The Bridge of your Nose
2. The Cheekbone, at the corner of the eye socket
3. The Forehead, anywhere on the eyebrow
4. The Lips, your Head Butt will Split them and break or loosen teeth

Remember; Every response you deliver must be with **Maximum** power. If you show any mercy at all you will most likely **Not Live** to regret it.

There is a Nerve or Pressure Point that if it is attacked correctly, it will set you Free. Here is a simple test to do with a friend on each other, GENTLY! One of you stands with your back flat against the wall. The other holds a regular pencil with one hand. Hold the pencil horizontally where the Nose meets the upper lip. Hold it firmly, but don't cause pain. The person against the wall slowly tries to lean or bend forward, gently.

The Headlock Hold: If the attacker has you in **a Headlock** (you can use this move to escape) in one smooth motion, Swing whichever arm is next to the attacker, up and over their shoulder. Placing the palm of that hand on their cheek, your middle (Social) finger goes under their nose. In a rearward motion, forcefully bend the attacker backwards; he will be forced to release you. As he falls, grab his crotch and get rough, give them a hammer blow to the diaphragm, a chop to the Adams Apple. If you can't reach the nose, reach the crotch from between the legs, grab their package and squeeze, jerk then squeeze again. Don't forget, you can grab the Ears. Then escape or continue to abuse them, with your new bag of tricks. Practice these moves slowly; they will become more natural.

Cheek Grab (The ones on the face) the cheek grab is another move that is more punishing than most. Your hand is in a similar position as when you poke out the Eyeball. But, Your Thumb enters the mouth between the teeth and the cheek. You then grasp the cheek in your fist and get as rough as you like. You now have the attacker's undivided attention, make it count. Any compassion at this point would be a grave mistake, for you. The other hand is grabbing or hitting their Adams apple, their Ears, poking them in their Eyes. All while you're kicking, kneeing or stomping their crotch; don't stop until you feel safe. Then, Get away from him, quick.

** **Note:** I realize the average person has a different outlook on life than those, like me, who have been trained to respond differently to violence. (Not as if you're surprised or as if you've burned your hand) but look at the violence and evaluate its level of intensity or its true level of danger. Then in an instant meet or exceed that violence (OAO). As an example; several years ago, I found myself in a very vulnerable situation. I went into a little neighborhood bar, thinking it looked like a nice quiet place to have a cold beer. As I sat at the bar drinking my second beer, a rather large and burly individual approached me. I saw him coming (at 15') and had evaluated his threat level long before he reached my position. (You'll develop this level of Awareness) Before he reached me, I remained seated, turned and made direct eye contact. He asked in a rather gruff manner, if I knew I was in their bar and only Bikers in their club hang-out there. (Here is where your training comes into play) Before he finished his question, I had made a few observations.
1. He was strong, about 35 yrs old, 6'2" tall and weighed about 250 lbs.
2. His clothes were pretty *ripe* (dirty)
3. He wore gloves with the fingers cut off and heavy biker boots
4. His hair and scruffy beard were long enough to grab
5. He appeared slow moving, not quick or athletic
6. He positioned himself 'full front' view and within my reach.
What were my options? (Think about what you have read, now apply it).

**You must train yourself to be aware of who or what is going on 360 degrees around you, including the level of threat. Think about this; the way you present yourself, increases or decreases the level of threat you'll receive. It also communicates to others, if you are seen as a threat, a neutral or as an easy victim.

More about this biker bar scenario later.

New Situation: You are attacked while asleep, under the covers in your own bed. Even though you're startled and scared you must force yourself to evaluate your situation, answer these basic questions. While struggling to get your legs from under the covers;

1. Am I being beaten, stabbed, held down, or smothered?
(If being smothered, turn your head to either side and breathe)
2. Where is his center of gravity, his balance point?
3. Is he on me, legs straddling me, standing next to me? (Visualize him)
4. What is he saying?

How you respond is very important. The reason you must find his center of balance is to decide how to get him off of you. Your legs are much stronger than your arms, so visualize how you are going to use them. If he is sitting on you, straddling your body, several options, arch your back; grab him with your legs.
* If your arms are being held down, violently arch your back as to throw him forward into the headboard or wall, moving your arms will help.
* If your arms are free, you can use any of the moves for the hands, hammer blow, fingers, and elbows. Target mainly the Eyes, Nose and Ears because you want to deliver as much pain as possible. A hard punch or slap to the temple, ear or side of the neck will affect his balance. Grab and pull the arm nearest the edge of the bed, while pushing with the other to throw him off the bed, attack with legs, reading lamp, clock what-ever. When you can get a leg free, try to push his head or torso back enough to sweep your leg up and in front of his chest. Then with as much power as you can muster thrust him off of you. Follow with your all out attack.
* Continue the relentless attack at his vital points, don't stop until you are safe, or he is un-conscious, then stopping is your option, I wouldn't, he may be faking..
* Then get up, deliver several damaging kicks to his throat, diaphragm or crotch.
* Then get out of the house, **Forget the Phone**, forget clothes, **Get out of the House**, find help anywhere else.

New Situation: Two-handed choke (From the Front, Standing)
The attacker is right in front of you. His arms are either extended or bent and both of his hands are on your throat. Relax, we can handle this. Look directly into his eyes with disgust. **Two things are happening in this scenario.** His thumbs are closing off your windpipe making breathing difficult.

While at the same time the rest of his hands (without his knowing) are restricting your Carotid Arteries on the side of your neck below your ears. This stops the blood flow to your brain and you'll pass out in 10 seconds or less. So you need to get his hands off of your throat.

Try this; Thrust both hands directly between his arms and into his eyes.

Or this; Let go of him, put your arms down to your sides. **Then**; Right arm swings in a **forceful extended arc** (like a ballerina on steroids) up and over his arms and continues in this arc as you rotate or turn your body with it. At the same time your Left hand has quietly grasped his wrists, as if to hold them in place. The arc of your arm and your body twisting motion loosens his choke hold and traps both of his arms under your right arm pit. Keep going bending him forward with you. Now, Full reverse, drive your right Elbow forcefully back into the attackers Face, Anywhere, Eyes, Nose, Temple or Throat, BUT, Hard enough to daze him or her. You can repeat the Elbow Thrust several times if you like. Don't forget to use as many of the other moves as the opportunity presents targets.

There is another option to the Frontal Choke. You have probably played kickball, soccer or football and know how to kick powerfully with a straight leg. It doesn't matter how close you are to the attacker, it's the force that counts. The attacker won't care if you kicked him in the nuts with you foot, your shin or your knee, he'll only know that it hurts more each time you kick him. Remember, your goal is to get away, if you play nice, you lose.

Leg Kicks: In some situations you may be able to deliver a side kick to the attacker's leg or knee. This is a very good way to disable a person of any size. The target is the knee joint itself either straight on or to the side of the joint. I prefer the side of the knee, as it has less protective tissue and is therefore easier to break. Your ability to deliver a damaging kick is easier than you might think.

A good example of how to deliver a leg kick is to watch the Participants on the MMA, Mixed Martial Arts Programs on TV. You'll also see examples of how to deliver many of the Strikes, Blows and Kicks, that I have introduced you to in this book. I don't want you to try to become an expert; I only want you to get a sense of the mechanics involved in the various deliveries.

Now that we have covered various situations and you have had time to think about my Biker Bar Scenario.

What would you have done in that situation?

You know I could easily drive the beer glass or mug into his face. Aiming at his eyes, nose and ear or mouth area. You know I could easily hit each of them at will. My follow-up would be a combination of the same tools you now have. But, since you are now more aware, consider the bikers 20' away, waiting and watching?

Here is his basic question again; He asked in rather gruff manner, if I knew I was in their bar and only club members hang-out there. My response went something like this; "No, I noticed a few nice bikes outside but, I didn't know it was a private bar. I just wanted a few quiet beers and as long as you guys hold it down, we'll be fine". I could tell by the look on his face my answer was not what he expected. He turned and walked over to his biker buddies, I could hear them talking. He soon returned to my side, I turned and looked him straight in the eye and I said, "Well?" He put a cold bottle of beer on the bar and said; "We have no problem with that".

This is a true story and it shows how far, "The way you present yourself to others, goes". Your self confidence and your carriage is something everyone can see and they will respond accordingly. That same large biker told me later that they were surprised that I did not show any fear of them or the situation. He went on to say that when we were face to face, he saw no fear in my eyes and that bothered him. My purpose in telling you my Biker story was to illustrate how important it is that if you truly believe in yourself. You can make a difference and become a Mental Force to be reckoned with. Nobody has the right to inflict their will on you. Your mind is your best, most powerful weapon and as you practice these moves and develop Attitude, you'll become even more of a Physical Force. Your new motto; *Attitude* is everything, say it often, believe it, I'm an old Marine, I still believe it.

Let's take a little time to summarize and pull all of this material, i.e. Your New Awareness and Defense Options, Together.

*Note: If you wear high heels, hold one in each hand and hit anything you can, as hard as you can with the heels.

Some things may have been overlooked, gone unsaid or not explained thoroughly. I want to clarify the purpose of this book is to give you the mental and physical tools you need to defend yourself, even save your own life or the lifes of others.

In the event you are attacked and it is obviously with the intent of raping you, you must be able to draw on your mental strength to calm yourself and think. I understand this is a tough situation and you didn't ask for it to happen. But, you'll get through it if you have the proper mindset. You can do anything even the unthinkable in a controlled crisis. Your thinking must be quick and clear, you must be able to anticipate events before they take place. You may have to appear to play along; your goal is to get the attacker or rapist to drop his or her guard. Initially you will have no control over what is going on and that is his or her entire perverse goal. Knowing what to expect will help you act the part of the helpless victim until you see your opportunity. Think back to my rapid assessment of the biker, you should be able to do that as well. Later, the police will need a description of the rapist. You know, the guy holding his eye in one hand and his crushed nuts in the other. If it gets to the point of actually having to perform sex acts your target list just got much shorter, do you remember remember my carrot analogy? Just Do IT! Remember, to hesitate is to lose everything. Do what you have to do to stay alive.

Do you need to justify your actions, no; you did what was necessary to stay alive. This person is in the act of defiling your body for some measure of perverse gratification, after which he will most likely kill you. How merciful is that? To show any concern as to how much damage you may or may not inflict on this degenerate is ridiculous. They are going to kill you when he, she or they are done having their way with your body (Alive or Dead). Your only goal is to stay alive you can later say, "Too bad I had to hurt someone".
Remember, when you can get away, get away! Don't stop to get dressed or find a cell phone, Get Out! In some area's people are so used to yelling, they ignore calls for help. Nobody ignores **"FIRE!"** **Attract attention, Get to Live Help!**

** The Second Greatest mistake is to have **quit fighting too soon, you lose.**
** The Greatest mistake would be to have not fought at all and now you're dead.

For those who are Joggers: What is your opinion of security?
Why do you run alone, do you feel safe, are you invincible?
If you are a jogger and must run alone in the woods, try this; carry a child's thick pencil or a contractor's flat red pencil you know, the big flat one. (A dull point on each end) Reason; both types of pencils are legal and lethal. Also, a short 10" piece of 1" dowel, taper the ends to a dull ¼" point, cover it with colored adhesive tape, it'll help you concentrate. ;-) or (an ounce of wood is worth a pound of cure).

There are numerous bad things that can happen to all of us. Our goal is to identify them as quickly as possible and if we're able, avert or minimize the damage.

Remember these basic elements and adjust them as you must for a comfortable fit.
1. Become more aware of your surroundings
2. Think positive, "I will not be a Victim" and I carry this little stick.
3. Watch people, identify any threats and note their body language or attitudes.
4. Visualize yourself in each of the situations. OAO

Find a serious friend to practice with a male if possible. You must practice to achieve a quicker and natural response. This will also help your Self Confidence.

Notes: (write down your thoughts and idea's you need to think about.)

Home Security is the next topic:

Home Security

Do you have any weapons in your home? The only correct answer is: YES!

Some of the most common items in your home can and should be considered weapons. I will teach you how they are to be used to defend you and your family. Many people have guns, but an alarming number of them haven't a clue about how to use them safely inside their home. That is why occasionally we hear of family members being shot and even killed by other family members.

Most guns found in the home are in either of two places. They are in a nightstand near the bed or in a desk drawer. Everyone knows that, even a Rapist or Burglar. But, these people are crooks some have their own guns, they are stolen of course. If they (the crooks) are already in your home when you come back, they have probably looked in both of your secret hiding places and have your gun. What now? Hide it somewhere else, close to where you're more apt to be when they break-in. You should make an attempt to be creative knowing your life is at stake.

Situation: For some reason you wake up and think someone is in your house. **Do not turn on the lights.** Quietly get your *loaded* gun and move to the darkest corner of the room and sit down on the floor (behind something). **Wait Quietly, Wait very quietly!** By doing this, you'll accomplish several things. You'll have time to decide if what you hear is **an intruder, a family member, the dog or cat.** (3 out of the 4 of these, you do not want to shoot).

If you have children, move to a point (a Dark Area) where the intruder must pass your position. Again, identify your target. When I say identify your target, **I mean Visually, Not Verbally.** Be sure, is this a family member or is it an intruder? Surprise is on your side, always work from the dark. If you are sure it is an intruder you have a legal right to shoot in the defense of your home and your family. There is no reason to get all excited and give away your position or your edge. Simply aim your loaded, cocked gun at the center of the mass and gently squeeze the trigger, **twice.** If the intruder still poses a threat, shoot again. If they are trying to leave, you make the call. I'd shoot them again; they broke into our house, to harm us. To be afraid is fine, use the fear to sharpen your senses. On the other hand, **panic is useless and your enemy will kill you.**

You can find reassurance in the fact that you know where everything is located in your home; this allows you to know where they are by what you hear. If you just moved into a new house or apartment, dim the lights and quietly move around to familiarize yourself. Then turn the lights off and move around, learn the layout. If you think it is too dark, place a few night lights in strategic spots. They'll light up any possible intruder hiding spots. Even well placed external lights can be used to illuminate darker interior areas.

** **Note:** Some intruders are on drugs looking for something they can sell or trade for dope. **Don't be Stupid or so arrogant you try to talk them into giving up. Remember, you and your family are the victims and they might shoot or stab you, even hurt your family or worse.** All your 'Sense of Fair Play' will accomplish is to give them the edge. Think about this; are you a witness to a crime? Could you send them to jail? **Don't become a social worker** at 3:00 AM to a Thief, who may kill you and rape your family members.

Now, I want you to think about what kind of weapons you have in your home or apartment. We've talked about guns and I'm sure you've already thought of the knives in the kitchen drawer. You may have also thought about the large Carving Fork. What else could be considered a weapon?

First, let's establish what you think and how you are going to use a weapon? Are you going to?
1. Swing it? Soap on a Rope
2. Throw it? Coffee mugs, dishes
3. Poke with it?
4. Stab with it?
5. Hammer with it?
6. Spray it? Any Aerosol spray (Wasp spray shoots over 20 feet, target; Face.
7. Flame on, with it? This endangers the house, but it could save you.
8. Shoot it? A pistol with laser sights, Grip lights laser, bullet impacts at dot.
9. A Hardwood walking cane is legal to carry anywhere. Swing, hit or jab.
10. A straight umbrella is also a good poking tool.

Which of these actions or choices sound like something you could do to stop an attacker, rapist or intruder from harming you or your family?
If you answered: All of them, Good you are correct.

These items are great, as you look around your home perhaps you'll think of more. Can you picture yourself actually defending yourself using household goods as weapons? Let me paint you another verbal picture. I will be standing-in as the potential victim, but I won't wear the frilly apron. This starts out in the Kitchen; **Ok, I am alone in the house**, working in the kitchen next to the sink. I'm emptying the dishwasher while watching the late news on TV. As I turned, some movement in the dark hallway just caught my eye. Something I had read told me, do not stand-up and don't turn until I have a weapon of some kind. So, with the dish towel in my left hand (the side the intruder is on) I firmly grasp the cast iron metal meat tenderizing hammer in my right hand. I can sense the slow, quiet and methodical approach of the intruder. The book said; I should time my turn so we'll be face to face as I am ready to strike. Hopefully, he'll be as scared and surprised as I am. Causing him to freeze, then, I'll beat him senseless.

Having read this book (Security for Today's Women) over and over, I know I have to throw the dish towel into the air towards the intruders face as a distraction. Then, I'll hit the sucker as hard as I can, wherever I can. (I can't wait to see how this plays out, can you?) Anyway, to make a long story short, I did what my new, favorite book told me to do.
(I'm safe) The dish towel covered his face just like the book said it would and I hit him, several times, from head to toe. The intruder spent three days in the hospital. (I'm sure He's very sorry) because when he came home, he was mad as hell. But, I'll bet he doesn't lock his keys in the car and climb in the bedroom window again. And, He'll think twice before trying to sneak in and scare me like that. Moral of the story: **It's better to be Safe than Sorry**, wouldn't you agree?

Sorry! Things were getting too gruesome. Eventually, you may be able to see the humor in my portrayal of a Modern, Aware and Awesome Woman with Attitude. (Sounds kinda like it could be my wife).

Authors note: There is nothing more attractive than an Intelligent Self assured Woman, who exudes Confidence, with just enough Attitude to add to her Mystic. (OMG!, So, you have you met my wife)?

Let's get back to the list of things you have or haven't thought of as possible weapons found in most homes. Your list may vary; the key is to keep an open mind. You'll soon be thinking of shopping in second hand stores and yard sales, as being at the proverbial neighborhood arms dealers.

Potential weapons: The everyday walking cane, (any variation), Broken Broom Handles-spear, Mop handles-spear, Ball Bats (wood or metal), Golf Clubs, Knives, Swords, Lamps, Paper weights, Statues, Vases, Belts with Buckles (a couple of wraps around your hand don't tie it, swing it hitting with the buckle) Heavy mugs, Fire Place end-irons. **Always target the Head, No EYES, can't catch you.**

Don't forget the multitude of aerosol sprays under your sink, the laundry room, or in the bathroom. Try this "Outside", Hold a fireplace lighter out at arm's length, light it, hold a spray can close to the flame but away from you, hair spray or paint closely, past the flame. Be Careful, you have a flame thrower. This also works well on wasp nests and poisonous spiders. Any type of spray will work; the target is the face, especially the Eyes. If he can't see you, he can't hurt you. Don't forget, he's the bad guy and wants to harm to you, 'so, do unto others, first'. **Do you want something you can carry around, even have it in your car or under your pillow?** Go to the market and get the pack of ivory soap bars, usually four bars to a pack. A doubled pair of knee high socks or nylons, put one sock inside the other and drop in one whole dry bar of ivory soap. Then tie a knot at the edge of the bar and two knots at the end. One knot holds the bar of soap in place; the other keeps it from slipping out of your hand. Practice by hitting a heavy pillow until you get used to its weight. This is known as **a Jailhouse Blackjack**; it will break bones, cave in heads and is a very serious **Close Quarters Weapon**.

How would you Summon Help?

Have you given much serious thought as to how you would summon help, if **you really need help Right Now?** The usual response is pretty matter of fact, "I'd just yell at the neighbor, they're good people". Great, Good idea, but they're staying at her mother's place in the Bronx this weekend. "Next, I'd call 911, the police", sorry cell phone is in the other room and the land line has been cut. How about a small hand held boat horn? They cost, 3 to 5 bucks and will wake the dead and scare the crap out of the intruder, even louder than a gun. If you hear someone rattling the door, get your gun, turn outside light on. **Don't go outside, call 911**

You Say,"This is -*Name*---, a man with a gun is trying to break into my house at --*Address*--. (**What**? How do you know he has a gun? Do you know he doesn't have a gun?). *The police will respond quicker to a call about a man with a gun, OK?*

You can DIY or have motion lights installed in strategic areas in your yard. They are nice when you drive up to your garage; the light comes on and stays on for a set amount of time. You can ask about them at any Lowe's or Home Depot store. They cost around $30.

There are other ways to sound an alert, put a whistle on your key chain or wrist band, with your pepper spray. The pepper spray is always good; you hold it at the ready when you walk to your car. When you unlock and open the car door, wait for the light to come on, if someone is in your back seat, spray them thoroughly, then slam the door and run, shouting for help.

As you review this material, please pay particular attention to how simple and straight forward the responses are. I have gone over them so many times and each time, I try to refine the moves to be more natural or fluid. The smoother, simpler the moves, the more apt you are to remember them. Should the need arise and you find yourself in a bad situation, make a special effort to calm yourself. Focus on the levels of danger and deal with the most intense first, in as direct and 'as matter of fact as possible'. You know you can do whatever is needed to meet and exceed the level of violence coming at you. Keep it as simple as, live or die.

Be Strong in your mindset, "I won't allow you to do this to me". One of the strongest thoughts (Mindsets) I ever learned was to "Mentally Refuse" to give the other person permission to hurt me in any way. There are many ways to reach a positive mindset, focus or meditative type of self awareness. Just try to think or concentrate on yourself and what you need to do to be safe and happy. You can take comfort in the knowing that as you think your way through this material, you are growing in both mind and spirit. Remember, if they try to mess with your mind or spirit, you know how to poke their eye out. ;-) So, is the pen indeed mightier than the sword? If you get up close and personal, use it! A metal pen is awesome and legal.

The intent of this material is not to advocate violence. It is intended to give nice people like you a fighting chance, when you are confronted by the uglier side of life.

Remember, Think, Stay Calm, expect to fight for your Life. Think of it as a matter of fact. Because turning the other cheek really hurts...
Look, Listen; Respond in kind, till it's done.

Have a safe day

*** Abused or Battered ***

Get out!! Call the local authorities or 911 now! If you hide abuse, it only gets worse. If you are being abused or battered by a family member, spouse, or lover, report them. To wait may cost too much. You are not alone a Woman is Battered every 15 seconds.

** I'm Sorry, but, if it is ongoing, this material cannot help you quickly enough, you need help now!! Call 911 Now!
They'll call a local women's shelter.
Please make the 911 call that can and will save your life.
Contact the Local Police or County Health Services.

The FOUR best things you can do are:
1. GET OUT (First GET AWAY, out of the reach of the abuser)
2. GET HELP from POLICE. CALL 911
3. GET HEALTHY (MENTALLY & PHYSICALLY)
4. GET A HAPPY LIFE, (Self Worth, Self Esteem, and Confidence)

You know in your heart you deserve better, but only you can change it.

* PLEASE, if you know someone who is being battered, pass this information on, help them anyway you can. What are good friends for?

Did you give anyone permission to treat you like this? You can take back your self esteem; there are several ways to reach out for help. The first step is to take control of your life and decide you've had enough. If you cringe or cower in fear you'll get what the abuser wants to give you, more abuse, less control of your life.

 It is my sincere hope you find it within yourself to muster the courage to reach-out. You know you deserve better, but you must reach-out to get help.

Intentionally left blank and for Emergency phone numbers and notes.
■ ■■■

Local contacts: Phone Numbers

Police Emergency 911
***

National Domestic Violence Hotline
1-800-799-7233
***

National Sexual Assault Hotline
1-800-656-4673

Use this page to write your thoughts and list the things you can and will implement into your life to make it safer, more enjoyable and hopefully longer.

The more you write, the more Confidence and Attitude you'll gain and the better your chances.